BODYWEIGHT TRAINING

Get Bigger, Faster, and Stronger with Calisthenics

Table of Contents

Introduction

Congratulations on downloading your personal copy of *Bodyweight Training.* Thank you for doing so.

The following chapters will cover the benefits of bodyweight exercises as well as beginner, intermediate, and advanced exercise routines. The first chapter will also cover how different you will be in just 12 weeks.

There are plenty of books on this subject on the market, thanks again for choosing this one! Every effort was made to ensure it is full of as much useful information as possible. Please enjoy!

CHAPTER 1

12 WEEKS

If we lived in a perfect world, we could lose weight and fat instantaneously. Unfortunately this isn't how our body works. Everything from the neurologic system to hormones can signal any change to your exercise routine and diet.

If you try to make a drastic change, like reducing calorie intake from 2,800 to 1,400 each day or take on an hour's worth of boot camp class at your first day back in the gym, the way your body chooses to adapt will do you more harm than good.

Your body will think that the food supply is short, you are beginning to starve, and it will start to save calories, and it will begin to burn protein to produce energy. This shuts down the way the body burns fat and causes the downward spiral that will end up causing metabolic damage. When you reduce calories, you are going to have to continue reducing calories. It's important that you stay away from this.

When you choose to try to reduce your intake of calories or your resting metabolic rate to lose weight fast, this will only cause rebound weight gain and not lasting weight loss. Around two-thirds of people who lose weight this way will end up gaining all the weight they lost back and then some extra within a four or five year period. The negative psychological impact that depriving yourself of food and pushing yourself during your workouts has on you isn't going to help you keep the weight off for any length of time.

If we look at the muscle and fitness side of this, diets that don't allow many calories can decrease the way your body is able to synthesize new, metabolically active muscle. This makes your workouts useless. It will only end up making your workouts feel harder because you have less energy.

It's important to understand that your muscles do not become stronger while working out. You become stronger and more fit in the days and hours between your workouts when the muscles begin to adapt and repair themselves. If you workout out for hours on end, or you're constantly working the same muscles groups, you're not allowing your muscles to recover. You're going to end up not seeing the results that you want. Nothing is more frustrating than working super hard and then not being able to reap any rewards.

Generally, many people should only aim to lose about two pounds each week so they can maintain lean muscle. It varies from person to person as to how fast they are able to lose weight.

For those of you that haven't gone to the gym in over a year, and are the farthest from your goal, the quicker you will reach your goal. Look at it this way: When you need to build more muscles and lose more weight, it will take less effort and time to challenge and improve your fitness.

When you start a new fitness routine, there are some people that will start noticing results before the pounds start coming off. This is due to the reduction of eating processed food, refined carbs, and sodium and leads to a noticeable change in bloating within just a couple of days. It isn't fat loss, but getting rid of the bloat gives a boost of motivation for most people. Significant muscle gain and weight loss take about eight weeks to set in.

However, the weight changes you experience aren't equivalent to all the benefits that are happing in your body. If you want to drop a significant about of fat and gain muscles, eight weeks may only show a difference in your upper arms. Local fat loss might actually be significant, but the increase in muscle keeps it from being noticed. For a person that starts an eight-week program to lose around 20 pounds, any gain in muscle will show as definition instead of bulk because there isn't as much fat anymore. A pound of muscle takes up more space than a pound of fat, so when people gain muscle while losing fat, they won't see as much of a reduction in body size.

For this reason, it is important that you pay attention, not only to your size and weight, but what your body fat percentage is to see a realistic look at how your body is changing. A lot of the scales out there now will measure your weigh and body fat. The improvements that you have with the strength and endurance of your cardiovascular system is going to be the best marker that you are becoming healthier.

If you ask a person why they don't work out, you will be hit with excuses like no time, not convenient, no membership, or don't understand how the machines work. Bodyweight exercises get rid of these obstacles. You just need a small space. It is relatively easy to squeeze in a workout wherever you might be. Exercising without equipment could also be a stress reliever if you are working at home or traveling.

Every decade of your life, will lose about six pounds of lean muscle. Research estimates that a person's metabolic rate will decrease around three to eight percent every decade after we turn 20. This is what causes the decrease in muscle mass. One of the best things that you can do to keep a strong metabolism and keep weight from adding up is to build more muscle mass. When you stress your body with heavy loads, you will become stronger. It doesn't matter if it is just your body, weight machine, or dumbbells.

It honestly couldn't get any easier when you use your own weight to build strength. You can customize it and do it anytime, anywhere. You don't need a gym membership or equipment and takes less than 30 minutes. If exercise machines, groups, treadmills, or free weights scare you, then your best bet would be bodyweight exercises so that you can get into a healthy routine.

So, how should you do bodyweight exercises? Cardio is beneficial, but building muscle is more important and is often overlooked. Doing quick cardio sessions like combining burpees in the middle of movements of strength like a set of lunges or pushups will keep the heart swelling while improving strength and muscle development. Very low, whole body aerobic training will improve fitness and muscle perseverance for females. Bodyweight exercises are one way to strength train. Research tells that lean muscle mass has a great effect on your blood vessels, brain, hormones, lungs and heart.

Different studies link various forms of strength training to these benefits:

- Reduces the risk of strokes, cardiovascular mortality, and acute coronary syndrome
- Increased resting metabolic rate
- Increased insulin sensitivity
- Removes metabolic waste from muscles during rest
- Reduced bone and joint pain
- Increased oxygen usage by muscles
- More energy
- Better sleep
- Lower stress level
- Healthy blood pressure
- Healthy cholesterol level
- More lean muscles

Another benefit of bodyweight exercises is they are able to

reverse the bad things that chronic dieting does to your body. You think that diets are meant to help the body. Yes, they are supposed to be helpful, but when somebody diets for years, they will often lose muscle tissue because of the low-calorie diet and the natural aging process. The low calories don't supply the right amounts of nutrients to keep the muscles strong. Muscles are essential to keep a healthy weight since they are metabolically active tissues that require more calories that fatty tissue needs.

How often should you train each week?

1. Perform exercises about two or three times each week. Each workout needs to use the big muscle group such as the core, chest, legs, and back to get the most out of the workout.

2. For every workout, try to do around eight or ten moves that work the muscles differently that you are working on. Perform each exercise in every set and perform eight to twelve reps of the exercise.

3. When you have completed your workouts, be sure to stretch about two to three days a week to keep from injuring yourself and to increase your range of motion, flexibility, and recovery.

It doesn't matter if your goal is weight loss or gain, just remember that you gain more benefits than how you look from bodyweight exercises. The following are different ways that bodyweight exercises are able to help your immune, hormonal, cardiovascular, and cognitive health:

1. It is a very productive workout. Research has suggested bodyweight-based exercises like plyometrics give wonderful fitness results with short periods. Plyometric training will improve the voluntary activation and endurance with concentric, isometric,

and eccentric contractions. Since there isn't any equipment, you can move from exercise to exercise more quickly so that you can reduce your rest time to maximize affects. You have heard about those brief but vigorous workouts that give big results. Eight weeks of conventional and high-intensity training improved fitness and reduced adiposity.

2. Helps to build and keep lean muscles. Building strength is an important part of keeping your metabolism strong as you get older because it increases your lean muscle mass that tends to decline as you age. Muscle mass plays an important part in maintaining metabolic functions and a healthy weight. It can help with hormonal balance, insulin sensitivity, and thyroid function. Your metabolic rate relies on how much lean muscle you have. This all means you are going to need extra calories to keep your weight.

    Have you ever noticed that muscular athletes are able to eat their weight in food? This is because they have to train for many hours every day and the muscles they have burn off more calories than fat does. Muscles are able to burn fat constantly, whether active or resting. Your growth hormone production increases with bodyweight exercises. People like to call your growth hormone the fountain of youth since they have fat burning abilities and help keep lean body mass.

    If you just like cardio workouts like swimming or running more than strength training, listen to this: Lifting weights will give you more strength and performance that provides power for different exercises. Building strength in the core or back is useful when you run or while strengthening the shoulders for swimming.

    Just a couple minutes of bodyweight training has a huge

effect on the metabolism of the body. You may have heard about the afterburn effect and know that when your exercising is finished that your body could still burn calories for many hours. Just doing a 45-minute exercise routine can increase your metabolic rate for up to 14 hours.

3. Improves heart health. Exercise makes the heart pump blood more efficiently. This will help your circulation and blood pressure. The heart becomes stronger just like any other muscle, when it has to work under pressure.

    Strength training is tied to getting healthier cholesterol levels which reduces the risk of strokes or heart attacks. Longevity is also associated with regular strength building exercises. Patients that have had heart attacks are told they should start doing weekly resistance training to build up their hearts' strength.

4. Reduces the risk for diabetes. Exercise can naturally help diabetes because it takes glucose from the blood. It tells the glucose to move into the muscles where it is stored as glycogen and used as energy later. It keeps glucose from building up in the bloodstream. Over time, a buildup of glucose can damage tissues, blood vessels, and organs.

5. Improves moods and fights depression. Exercise is often referred to as a natural Prozac because it helps to reduces stress and improves self-esteem, emotional health, sleep, confidence, and the ability to solve problems. Endorphins are released when you exercise, and that causes a natural lift in your mood. It can help with depression and improve energy levels naturally.

6. Helps to maintain cognitive function. When you exercise, you reduce DNA damage because of the anti-

aging effects of muscles and longevity. BDNF, a hormone, is stimulated when you exercise. This will then help your brain cells to regenerate. Exercise will lower inflammation and oxidative stress that is tied to disorders such as dementia and Alzheimer's.

7. Improves the health of bones and joints. Increasing the muscle mass will protect bones and joints, since strong muscles mean that you don't have to rely on your joints when you move. Exercising is able to help pain you may have in your hips, ankles, knees, and back while also increasing your bone density and strength. Exercising also helps to protect your frame and increase how you body fortifies bone reserves. This is critical to help prevent fractures, falls, and bone loss as we get older.

   Not everybody that exercises regularly ends up with sore muscles and joints that aren't flexible. Bodyweight exercises are able to help with flexibility and strength. When you use your full range of motion in bodyweight exercises, you are allowing your joints to move freely. It also helps to improve your posture and can reduce injuries due to exercises.

8. You will gain strength in your core. Your core is not just your abs. 29 muscles make up the torso, and simple movements are able to engage them all. You won't get tighter abs with these movements, but your posture will improve. It can also relieve lower back pain, and improve your overall performance.

9. It is challenging for any level of fitness. Bodyweight exercises are easily modified to make them easier or harder to perform. Just by adding more reps, doing the exercises slower or faster, taking shorter or longer breaks, or adding movements like clapping after every pushup, are ways to make an easy workout a bit tougher. With each modification, the progress is

obvious.

10. Your balance will become better. With this type of training, if you can increase your resistance means that you will increase your balance, as well. A normal squat can be made harder by doing a pistol, or single-leg squat. Movements such as that can help balance by increased control and body awareness.

11. You won't be bored. It is easy to get stuck in a rut with bench presses, lateral pull-downs, bicep curls, and treadmills. This is why bodyweight training is so exciting: There are numerous variations that could mix up any routine. Working with different exercises doesn't just relieve boredom, it's able to create progress and break through plateaus.

12. Changing and exercise is super easy. Exercising indoors isn't for everybody. Good news, you are able to do this alone, with a friend, inside, or outside. Add some strength moves to your next run in the park. Finish a swim in the pool with a bodyweight circuit to shake things up.

13. It helps prevent injuries. Injury is the main reason people stop working out. Preventing injuries is the top priority. Bodyweight training is safer for everybody. It doesn't matter their fitness level, age, or experience. Many movements could be effective for rehabilitation, even if you suffer from impairment. Bodyweight supported gait walking and training in stroke patients has been very effective with their rehabilitation.

Bodyweight Exercises Versus Weight Machines

The main reason that most women avoid weight training is it seems intimidating. Weight machines or free weights will provide you with the exact same benefits as bodyweight exercises because it all builds strength. But they require you to buy equipment and have knowledge of the equipment in order to use it properly. This sometimes means hiring a trainer. It is believed that weight machines don't allow you to use your full range of motion and only works one muscle group at a time. When you use free weights with bodyweight exercises it helps to work more muscles at the same time.

Bodyweight exercises are more accessible to the new strength trainer because they are modifiable and convenient. All you will need is space and your body to perform them. They are simple enough to do without supervision and still be safe from injuries. It's more forgiving when you use your body and gives you the ability to adjust your workouts to your ability as compared to using machines or free weights.

A lot of women are afraid of lifting weights because they think it will end up making them look masculine. You may be afraid that by focusing on strength training instead of burning calories will cause you to bulk up. That's not true. The female body will get leaner, stronger, and more toned. Women don't gain muscles like mean do. Most of the time, the female body will become tighter and smaller when they add strength training to their workout routine. Fat will be lost and the muscle they gain will take up less space than the fat did, even though it does weigh more.

What about cardio workouts that are aimed towards calorie burning? How do they stand up to strength or bodyweight training?

Building muscles help to speed up your metabolism, cardio exercises don't have that effect. If you do too much cardio work without proper rest, it can actually slow down your metabolism. Long cardio sessions can cause joint damage oxidative stress. This can lead to illness, pain, and injuries. Steady-state cardio such as cycling, swimming, or running helps to improve stamina, heart health, and endurance while cutting down on stress. If used with strength training, it can cause muscle wasting caused by overtraining or aging.

This has the ability to depress the immune system and cause an increase in cortisol levels, which inflames the body. Research has found that adults who do cardio regularly, like runners, could maintain fitness from aerobic activity. They can also lose some muscle from the areas that aren't trained. With a runner, their muscle will likely not change and they will only be able to carry strength in their legs. The muscle mass in their arms and core will decrease.

Long-term cardio might have other effects with time like neurotransmitter function, altering hormone levels, bone loss, or joint wear-out. Is there something better? Sure, build up the muscles in the entire body, but prevent injuries, burn-out, or boredom by changing bodyweight or strength training with cardio workouts.

Can You Lose Weight By Using Bodyweight Training?

Short answer, yes and no. Everybody will respond differently when they start to exercise. Things like sleep, stress levels, and diet all have an effect on determining if you will or will not lose weight fast or at all. Adding in bodyweight exercises to your normal routine can provide you with better results than cardio alone. They will end up making you leaner than not exercising.

Research has found that steady-state cardio has a lower fat-burning and metabolic potential than strength-training does.

Muscle growth helps with fat metabolism and is able to lower your cortisol levels. Cortisol is typically higher in people that are always stressed. Insulin is repaired when you lower your cortisol levels, and this will boost your body's natural fat-burning abilities. Also, you may be able to get a handle on your cravings and food intake when you build strength instead of only burning calories.

When you over train on cardio workouts, it will likely cause you to become hungry. This tells us that long aerobic exercises can work against weight loss. Research has found that many people tend to eat more to compensate for the calories they are burning, but they found that strength training doesn't have that effect.

Even if you do become hungry while building muscles, your muscles need more calories to help them grow. A woman with more muscle tone will develop an hourglass figure by adding shape to the legs and glutes, slim the waist, and tighten the stomach. Even though bodyweight exercises don't create a huge reduction on the scale, they are going to change how you feel and look.

Eating enough to sustain body weight while exercising will help to prevent your body from going into starvation mode. Starvation mode happens when you create a calorie deficit while losing weight. The negative side effect of eating less and exercising more is that if you are stressed out plus you are exercising a lot, the body will likely slow down the thyroid. When the thyroid works slowly, you will have difficulty maintaining your weight because your thyroid hormones play a crucial part in your metabolism.

How to See Results Quickly

Use the following steps to help safely speed up your weight loss goals.

1. Intensify your workouts and increase protein intake. The combo of increased protein and exercise will help you to build muscle and burn fat while you cut calories. You can reduce your calorie intake as well as increasing

your protein, so you won't lose muscle mass during your weight loss.

2. You must eat to give your body fuel. Every person needs different amounts of calories. Caloric deficits mean you burn more calories than you take in, which leads to weight loss, but a large deficit can create fat retention. A caloric surplus means you are eating a larger amount of calories than you burn, which is an ideal condition to build muscles. Don't get hung up on doing caloric math but just look at food as fuel. Pay attention to your body so that you know when it's hungry and eat whole foods that will fill you up on fiber, prevent fat storage and too much insulin secretion, and get you to your fat-loss goal.

3. Make strength training a priority over traditional cardio. Strength training is able to increase your calorie burn, even while you are resting, for 72 hours after you stop your workout. It also boosts the metabolism.

4. Recover. Give yourself a complete day each week to rest. Don't train the same muscles twice in a three-day period. Change up your intensity and workouts so that your body is able to recover. It is normal to feel sore between one and two days after your workout, especially when you are just starting, but you should not feel like you can't walk or move.

5. Change things around every six to twelve weeks. To keep your body from hitting plateaus and adapting, you need to vary your workout. This might mean changing your rep sets, taking a spin class a few times a week, or doing a different swim stroke. If you don't, your body may adapt to the workout so much that it won't receive any benefits from it.

CHAPTER 2:

BEGINNERS

Do the words dragon flags, pistol squats, and one-armed pushups sound scary to you? Maybe you don't have any experience with bodyweight or strength training and you're looking for some place to start. That's what we're going to cover in this first chapter.

When you don't have any experience with any sort of exercise programs, the important thing is to create a new habit of exercising. Bodyweight training may be one of the easier and simplest ways to exercise; there is a little bit of an infrastructure that you have to establish.

1. Come up with a routine.

2. Figure out how you want to track your progress.

3. Schedule times to work out.

4. Figure out where you are going to work out.

I'm going to try to help you work through all of these. Number two is easy, all you really need is a notebook that you keep with you when you workout. Three and four you will have to figure out completely on your own. Number one should be easy after you finish this book. All you have to do, really, is pick the workouts you like the best and do them at least three times a week.

For the best results, try to workout at the same time and in the same place. This place and time should be an easy choice. This means that you should pick an area that is most convenient. This could be at home, at a park, or at a gym. The only equipment that will show up in the workouts is a jump rope, pull up bar, dip bars, and a chair. The jump rope and chair are easy, for the other two, you can come up with alternatives or purchase one. Make sure you also pick the time that is most convenient. For the most part, you're only going to work out for 30 minutes, three times a week.

Are you able to wake up 30 minutes earlier to work out first thing in the morning? And are you actually going to work out each morning? You have to be completely honest with yourself. If you can't work out in the morning, that's perfectly fine. Everybody dreams of being that person that wakes up bright eyed and bushy tailed ready to do jumping jacks and sit-ups, but that's not the truth.

I have personally tried to do morning workouts, but after a few days, I stopped. It's not for me. I do better at night. Make sure you don't make it optional. Don't ask "should I exercise?" Tell yourself you're going to and view it as an appointment.

As a newbie, you are able to mix together simple moves to create a significant routine. You don't have to do anything fancy as a beginner to see the results.

There are four main moves that, even if you are an intermediate, give you the best results.

- Supermans

- Squats

- Bodyweight Rows

- Pushups

These four moves will train your pulling and push strength, work your legs, and help your posterior stability.

You're probably wondering why there isn't a core exercise listed. That's because when you perform these moves with correct form, you will be working your core muscles.

Also, don't worry if you can't do a pushup or some of the other moves. When you start out, begin with an easier or modified version of the exercise.

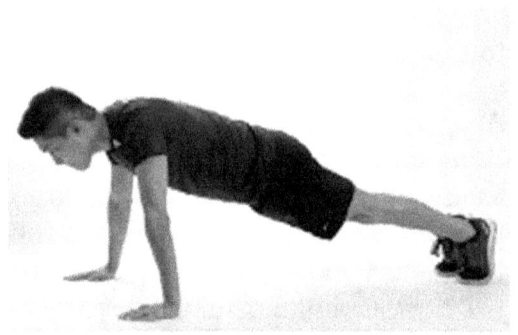

If you're not able to do a pushup, choose an elevated surface to place your hands on. This could be just a few blocks, the back of your couch, or the wall. Make sure it's not too easy though, it does need to be a

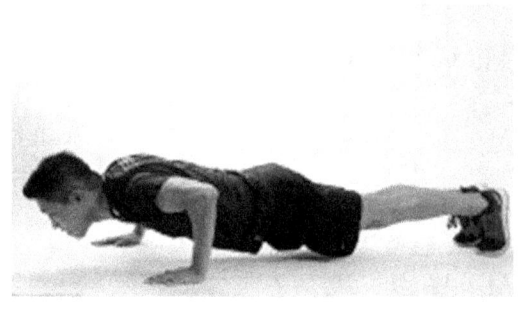

challenging, but you need to be able to perform it properly. If you find regular pushups too easy, elevate your feet. Place your feet on some blocks to increase the difficulty. Make sure that you always have your body in a straight line whenever you are doing a pushup, no matter if you have your hands or feet elevated. Elbows also shouldn't flare out but should be close to your body.

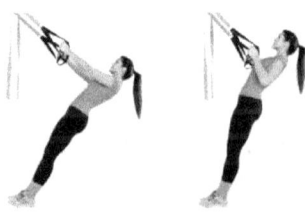

Bodyweight rows look like a horizontal pull up. You can use rings or pull up bar. With your feet out, and gripping the bar, pull your chest towards the bar. If you find a regular bodyweight row too hard, pick a higher bar. If you find them too easy, then you should try elevating your feet. Your body should also be in a straight line when performing this exercise.

For squats, all you do is squat down as if you are going to sit in a chair; making sure your knees stay above your ankles. If regular bodyweight squats are too hard, try sitting on a bench or chair and then immediately stand back up. Once regular squats get too easy, start doing ass-to-grass squats, and when that gets easy, do prisoner squats.

If those squats become easy, try doing Cossack squats. Some people confuse these for side lunges, but there is a big difference. For a Cossack squat, start by doing a side lunge and then lower over further, your calf and hamstring should touch. Do every rep on one side and then do it on the other side.

For the superman exercise, lay on your stomach and engage your lower back muscles and lift your legs and arms up off the ground. If this is too hard, spread your arms and legs to the side as far as you can. With supermans, you typically hold 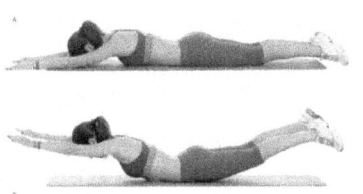 it for as long as you can. There are some workouts, though, that tell you to do a certain number of reps.

The secret to success is progressing your workouts. When something gets easy, don't just do more reps; make it a little bit harder. Those people that you see doing handstand pushups aren't just superhuman; they worked their way up to that.

Beginner Moves

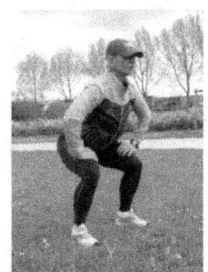 **Squat:** Start in a standing position with your hands out in front or behind your head. Start to push hips backward and squat down as low as you can go. Your knees should not move

21

forward or backward. Once you squat down, push yourself back up. The weight should be located in your heels and not your toes. Variations of the squat are sumo: where you have you legs positioned about shoulder width, and plie: where your legs are shoulder width apart, and your feet turned out.

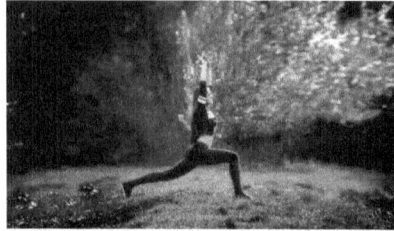

Pull Up: Stand at a pull up bar or rings. Grasp the bar or rings with hands, palms facing forward. Engage your muscles and pull yourself up until your chin is above the bar.

Lunges: Standing, with your arms by your side, step forward with your right leg and lower down. The front knee should stay above the ankle and never move forward. The back knee should move straight towards the ground.

Oblique Reaches: Lay on the ground with feet flat on the floor and hip width apart. Extend your arms by your side and lift your head slightly. Engage your oblique muscles and bend to touch your right fingers to your right heel, straighten, and repeat on the other side.

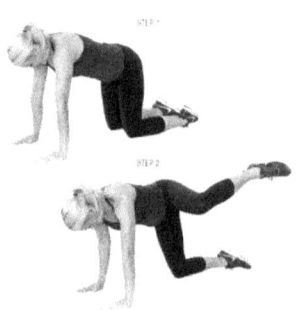

Fire Hydrant: Begin on your hands and knees. Raise one leg sideways, keeping your leg bent at a 90 degree angle.

Bird Dogs: Begin on hands and knees. Reach opposite arm and leg, bring back down, and repeat with the other side.

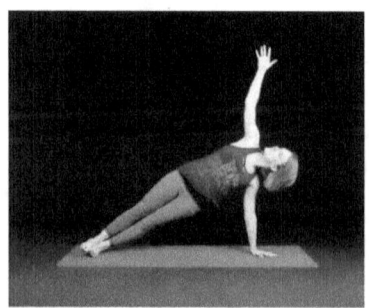

Side Plank: On one side, raise yourself up onto your forearm. The elbow should be directly beneath the shoulder. The legs should be stacked. The body should form a straight line.

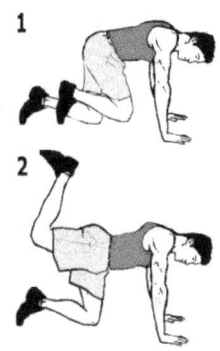

Donkey Kicks: Begin on hands and knees. Raise one foot up towards the ceiling, keeping your knee bent at a 90 degree angle. Lower the leg back down and repeat.

Fingers to Toe Lifts: While standing, lift your right foot to your left hand and touch your fingers to the foot. Bring the foot back down and repeat on the other side.

Pulse Ups: Lying on your back, lift your legs straight up with your feet towards the ceiling. Gently pulse your feet towards the ceiling.

Windshield Wipers: Lying on your back with your arms straight out to the sides. Raise your legs up with your feet pointing towards the ceiling. Lower the legs down to the right, raise them back up, and then lower them to the left, repeat.

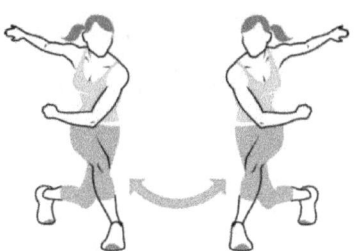

Speed Skaters: From standing, jump to the right and bring your left foot behind you and your left arm across your chest. Repeat this to the left.

CHAPTER 3

BEGINNER EXERCISES

100 Workouts

This workout looks harder than it is. You will be doing 100 reps, and you only have to do one set.

20 Leg Raises: 2 sets of 10

20 Crunches: 2 sets of 10

20 Tricep Dips: 4 sets of 5

20 Pushups: 4 sets of 5

20 Jump Squats: 2 sets of 10

Basic

Depending on your skill level, perform two to four sets of this workout. Try to keep from rest between exercises, but take a 60-second rest after each set.

50 Jumping Jacks

25 Squats

15 Pushups

30 Lunges, 15 on each side

30 Bicycle Crunches

60 Second Plank

Easy Full Body

Each exercise will provide you with how many sets you need to do before you move onto the next workout. Rest for a couple of minutes between each individual exercise, try to avoid resting between exercise sets, though.

40 Jumping Jacks, 1 Set

20 Squats, 2 Sets

8 Walking Lunges, 2 Sets

15 Crunches, 2 Sets

15 Knee Pushups, 2 Sets

20 Lying Oblique Reach, alternating sides, 2 Sets

30 Second Plank, 2 Sets

25 Fire Hydrants, 2 Sets

20 Bird Dogs, alternating legs, 2 Sets

30 Side Leg Lifts, each side, 2 Sets

25 Second Side Plank, 2 Sets

Five Minute Workout

This is a quick workout when you only have five minutes to get a workout in. Do three sets of this workout.

10 Knee Pushups

45 Second High Knees

10 Squats

10 Minute Workout

When you have a few extra minutes in your day, throw in this workout to get your blood pumping. Do this circuit three times.

1 Minute Cross Punches

10 Glute Bridges

1 Minute Hamstring Curls, alternating legs

10 Tricep Dips

15 Minute Workout

To get a better cardio workout, try this workout when you have 15 minutes. Do four sets of this circuit.

30 Second Forearm Plank

1 Minute Side to Side Shuffle

20 Forward Lunges, alternating legs

1 Minute Pivot and Reach

20 Minute Workout

For a full workout, and to really get your blood pumping, try this one out for size. Do five sets of this circuit.

20 Knee Pushups

1 Minute Curtsy Lunge

20 Lying Leg Curls, alternating legs

1 Minute Jumping Jacks

Butt Lifting Workout

For this exercise, you will be focusing on your glute muscles. Perform three sets of this circuit.

8 Modified Pistol Squats

8 Pulsing Plie Squats

8 One-Legged Plank Bridge, each leg

8 Supermans

8 Donkey Kicks, each leg

Cardio and Core

Perform the exercises as they say. Do all the sets for one exercise before moving to the next. Take a two-minute break between individual exercises.

60 Second Jump Rope, 3 Sets

40 Second Crunches, 3 Sets

30 Second Pulse Ups, 3 Sets

60 Second Fingers to Toe Lifts, 3 Sets

60 Second Standing Mountain Climbers, 3 Sets

30 Second Lying Oblique Reach, 3 Sets

45 Second Inchworm, 3 Sets

30 Second Superman, 3 Sets

20 Second Side Plank, each side, 3 Sets

Sweet At Home

There are three circuits in the workout. Repeat each circuit twice and then move onto the next circuit. Rest 30 seconds between each circuit set, and two minutes between each circuit.

Circuit One

> 20 Squats
>
> 20 Pushups
>
> 20 Jumping Jacks

Circuit Two

> 60 Second Plank with Alternating Leg Lift
>
> 15 Tricep Cips
>
> 20 Lunges

Circuit Three

> 20 Bicycle Crunches
>
> 30 Second Wall Sit
>
> 15 Squat Jumps

Toned and Cardio

Each exercise will be performed in three sets. Perform all sets before you move onto the next exercise. Rest a minute between each exercise.

> 60 Second Inchworm, 3 Sets
>
> 30 Second Side Plank, each side, 3 Sets
>
> 60 Second Standing Side Crunches, 3 Sets
>
> 60 Second Russian Twist, 3 Sets

45 Second Spiderman Plank, 3 Sets

30 Second Donkey Kick, each side, 3 Sets

45 Second Windshield Wipers, 3 Sets

45 Second Crunches, 3 Sets

60 Second Crab Kick, 3 Sets

45 Second Shoulder Taps, 3 Sets

5 – 10 – 15

For this workout, you will repeat the whole circuit five times

5 Pushups

10 Sit Ups

15 Squats

10 Second Rest

5 Jump Squats

10 Alternating Lunges

15 Reverse Crunches

20 Minute HIIT

Repeat each circuit three times before you move onto the next circuit. Rest for a minute between each circuit.

Circuit One

30 Second Jump Squats

10 Second Rest

30 Second High Knees

10 Second Rest

Circuit Two

>30 Second Pushups

>15 Second Rest

>1 Minute Wall Sit

>15 Second Rest

Circuit Three

>30 Second Mountain Climbers

>10 Second Rest

>30 Second Jump Lunges

>10 Second Rest

Hear Pumper

You only have to do this workout in one set.

>10 High Knees, each leg

>2 Star Jumps

>5 Plank Jacks

>10 Mountain Climbers

>20 Butt Kickers, each leg

>15 Second Jump Rope

>1 Burpee

>20 Speed Skaters

>1 Squat Jump

>10 Jumping Jacks

Beginner Butt

Each exercise in this workout should be done four times. Rest for two minutes before moving onto the next exercise.

15 Squats

30 Donkey Kicks

30 Fire Hydrants

30 Second Wall Sit

15 Bridges

30 Side Leg Raises

Legs and Core

This is probably the hardest beginner workout, but you have complete control over this one. Begin by setting a six-minute timer and try to do as many sets of the first three exercises as you can. Try to rest as little as possible between each exercise. Then set another six-minute timer and do the same for the last three exercises. Make sure you don't start out going too fast. Otherwise, you are going to get winded earlier on and struggle to finish. Go at a steady pace, and if you feel like you can speed up, then do so.

10 Forward Lunges

15 Mountain Climbers, each side

10 Sumo Squats

10 Side Lunges

15 Shoulder Tap Planks, each side

10 Burpee

CHAPTER 4

INTERMEDIATES

We have talked about the benefits of bodyweight exercises. You don't need any equipment. Bodyweight workouts can improve power, speed, athletic performance, burn fat, and build muscle. By adding a jumping element you take the intensity up a level and it becomes a plyometric move.

Plyometric training isn't intended for newbies or anyone that has recently experienced an injury. You need to have good form and focus when performing these exercises. That's why it's important to do these types of workouts before you tire and your performances slacks.

If you've never done a plyo workout before, you should only focus on three or four exercises first in your workout after your warm-up. Perform two to three sets with three to five repetitions in each set. Do this at least two but no more than four times each week. Give yourself two to three days to between plyo sessions. Even if you cannot do all of that, you will still receive some of the plyo benefit. Training moderately with plyometrices a couple of times a week is effective in creating strength and power. Remember, you don't have to purchase anything special for this.

Intermediate Moves

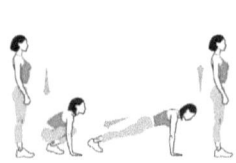

Plyo Pushup: Perform your regular pushup, but when you push back up, add more strength so that your hands come up and you clap before coming back down. If you can't do it in full pushup, then try it in a modified pushup position.

Squat Thrusters: Begin in high plank, move your feet forward into a wide squat and bring your hands into a prayer pose. Make sure your back stays straight, keep your shoulders down, and the chest out while you are in the squat position. Pause and then bring your hands back to the ground and jump back into the high plank. Do this as quickly as you can.

Plyo Lateral Lunge: Stand with your feet together and your arms by your side. Engage your abs, send back your hips, and take a right step with your right foot. Bend the right knee while keeping the left leg vertical while you lower into a lunge. To help your balance, place your hands out to the side or in prayer position. In one move, push with your right foot and hop to where your left was and send the left leg out to the side and into a lunge on the left side. If it helps, picture it as a side step with a hop. Repeat, alternating sides each time.

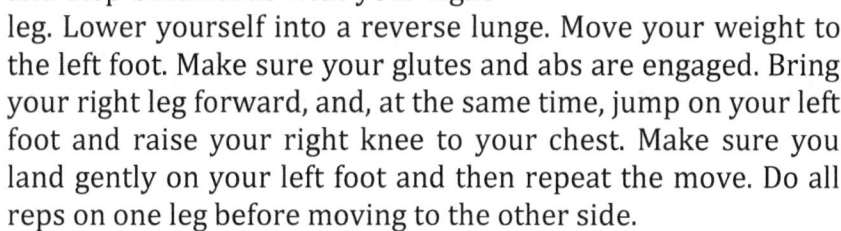

Reverse Lunge with Knee-Up: Place your feet as wide as your hips and step backwards with your right leg. Lower yourself into a reverse lunge. Move your weight to the left foot. Make sure your glutes and abs are engaged. Bring your right leg forward, and, at the same time, jump on your left foot and raise your right knee to your chest. Make sure you land gently on your left foot and then repeat the move. Do all reps on one leg before moving to the other side.

Box Drill: This move works the calves. Begin standing on your right foot with the knee bent slightly. You arms should stay loose at your side so that you can keep your balance. Hop to the right, staying on the right foot. Staying on your right foot, hop to the left. Now hop to the front and then to the back. Switch to the left leg and reverse the direction. Try to do quick and small jumps. For an easier variation: Do this exercise with both feet and try to build more speed as you jump.

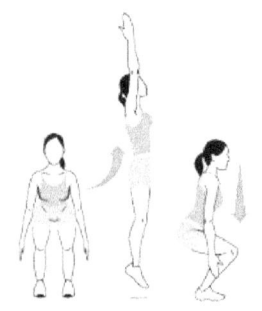

Frog Squat Jump: Place you feet slightly wider than hip width and turn out your toes. Drop into a deep squat and allow your hands to touch the floor. Jump up like a frog would. Keep your landing on the balls of you feet and repeat this movement as quickly as you can, and try to get higher each time.

Long Jump: Place your feet hip width apart. Crouch down into a squat with your arms behind you. Jump forward with your feet together, swinging your arms so that you keep your balance and land on your feet with your knees slightly bent. If you have the space, continue to jump forward, or turn around and then jump back to where you were. Try not to rest between jumps.

Burpees with a Tuck Jump: Perform a normal burpee. Once standing, don't perform the normal jump. Instead, bring your knees up as high as you can and tuck the knees towards your chest. Land softly and continue into your next burpee.

Alternating Lunge Jumps: Begin by stepping forward with your right foot into a low lunge. Engage your abs and keep your right knee above the right ankle. 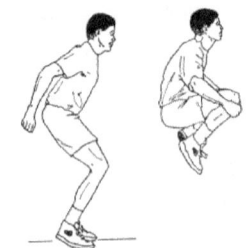 Shift all of your weight to the right foot and jump. Switch your leg position while in the air so that you land with your left foot in front and the right foot in back. Drop back into a low lunge and repeat. Think about height not speed.

Tuck Jumps: Place your feet shoulder width apart. Keep your knees bent and your hips back. Jump as high as possible and bring your knees up to your chest. Land softly on toes in the starting position. Keep jumping and avoid resting if you can.

Judo Roll with Jump: While lying on your back, tuck your knees into your chest with your ankles crossed. Engage your abs and roll yourself up into a seated position and rest your left foot on the ground. Using your core, come to a standing position on your left foot. Lower yourself back to the start position and switch your feet. For a modified version: Push yourself up with your hands and get your balance before jumping up. You can also use both feet to do the jump up.

Kneeling Jump Squat: Start by kneeling with legs spread slightly wider than your hips. Take your arms behind you and swing them to the front to help you get the momentum to jump to a squat position on both feet. Step the right foot backwards to come down onto your right knee. Bring your left foot back so that you are on both knees and then lower yourself back to the starting position.

Full-Body Plyometric Pushup: This is doing a regular pushup except your elbows are at a 90-degree angle. Push up as hard as you can so that you are momentarily floating. Keep the core tight, so your hips don't drop as you land back into a high plank. Continue onto the next rep. To modify this: Master the plyo pushup that we covered earlier.

Single-Leg Deadlift into Jump: Stand on your left leg with you knee bent. Bend forward at the hips and let the right leg move up behind you until the right leg and chest are parallel to the floor. In a single movement, swing your arms forward, let your chest rise, and push off the floor with your left foot. Move your right knee to your chest. Gently step with your left foot and quickly lower back into the bent over position. Make sure you keep your right foot off the ground the whole time. To make this easier: After you have landed, tap your opposite toe on the ground to help maintain your balance. You can also place your fingertips on the ground while your leg is behind you.

Horizontal Jump to Tuck Jump: Place your feet together. Bend your knees slightly and then push of the ground, jumping to the right as far as you can. When you land, do a tuck jump. Now push off again and jump to the left. When you land, jump into a tuck jump. Repeat and alternate sides.

Pistol Squat Roll with Jump: Stand on your left leg with the knee slightly bent, and your right foot off the ground and stretched in front of you. Balance your weight on your left foot, engage your core, rotate the hips back and slowly lower yourself into a low pistol squat. For your balance, extend your arms forward. Hold yourself in the squat. Drop your butt to the ground and rock slightly on your back. Roll your weight back onto your left foot and stand, jumping as high as you can. Softly land and repeat.

Plyometric Pushup to Squat: Begin in a normal pushup position. Push up has hard as you can and generate some momentum. When you raise up, tuck your knees into your chest and take your feet under your body. You should be in a deep squat. Hold for a moment and then jump into a pushup and repeat.

Side to Side Shuffle: With knees slightly bent, shuffle to the right about three steps then shuffle to the left. Repeat this for a time.

Inchworm: Begin by placing your hands on the ground in front of your feet. Walk your hands out into a plank position, and then walk your feet up to your hands. Without standing, walk your hands back out and repeat.

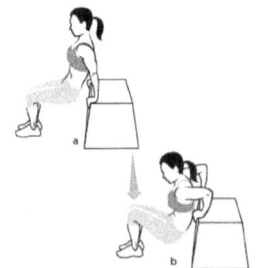

Scissor Skier: Begin by standing, arms at your side. Jump into a high lunge with the opposite arm raised to the leg in the front. Jump again, alternating the arms and legs.

Tricep Dips: Sit on the edge of a chair or other hard surface. Slide your legs out in front of you with your heels resting on the ground. Push yourself up and off the chair, and lower yourself down in front, as low 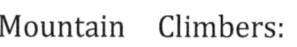 as you can. Push back up and repeat.

Bridges: Begin by laying on your back and your feet flat on the floor. Engaging your glutes, push your butt off the ground, and form a straight line with your body. A variation is to extend one leg and only push off the ground using one leg.

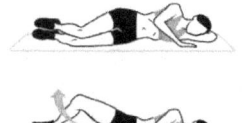

Clamshells: Lying on one side, stack your legs with your knees bent at a 45 degree angle. Rotate the hip on top to raise the knee off of the bottom. Lower and repeat.

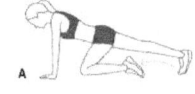

Mountain Climbers: Begin in a plank position. Quickly move your knees towards your elbows, alternating between legs.

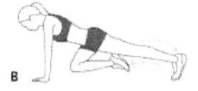

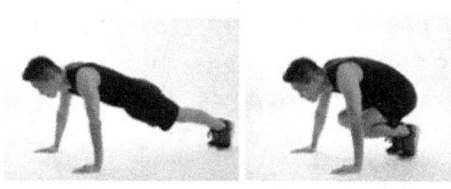

Plank Jacks: Begin in a forearm plank position. Step one foot to the side and then bring it back to the center, repeat with the other leg. Continue alternating the legs.

Burpees: From standing, bend over touching the ground, jump back to a plank position, jump your feet back to your hands,

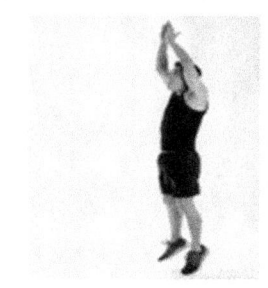

and stand. Repeat.

Bicycle Crunches: Lying on your back, raise your legs and shoulders slightly off the ground. Draw opposite knee to opposite elbow and start alternating, like you were peddling a bicycle.

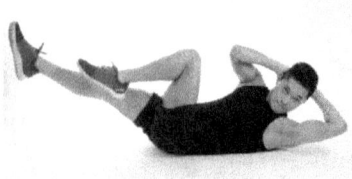

Russian Twist: Sitting on the floor, extend your legs out until you knees are at a 45 degree angle. Lean back slightly, engaging your abs, and rotate your torso from side to side.

Shoulder Taps: Start in a plank position and reach with your right hand to touch your left shoulder, bring your hand back down and repeat with the other.

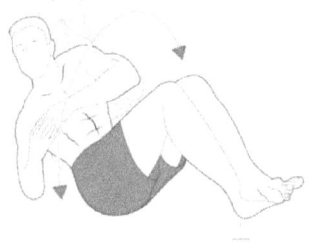

Touchdowns: From standing, jump into a squat position and

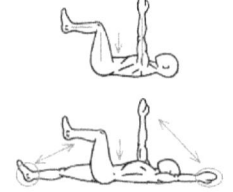

reach with one hand to touch the ground. Come back up and repeat with the other hand.

Dead Bug: Begin by lying on your back with hands pointing towards the ceiling and your legs bent at 90 degrees. Lower opposite leg and arm towards the floor. The arm should extend behind your head. Bring back up, and repeat with the other side.

CHAPTER 5

INTERMEDIATE EXERCISES

200 Workout

In this workout, you will be performing a total of 200 reps. There isn't any need for you to do more in the one set unless this felt too easy.

40 Leg Raises: 2 sets of 15 (one of each leg), 1 set of 10 (five reps on each leg)

40 crunches: 2 sets of 20

40 triceps dips: 4 sets of 10

40 pushups: 2 sets of 15, 1 set of 10

40 jump squats: 2 sets of 20

Sculpt Your Body Workout

Each exercise will tell you how many sets you have to do before moving onto the next. Try not to rest between sets of individual exercises. Rest 30 seconds to a minute between each exercise.

60 Second Butt Kicks, 3 Sets

45 Second Side Lunge, 3 Sets

30 Second Side Plank with Front Kick, 3 Sets each side

45 Second Speed Bag Punches, 3 Sets

60 Second Side to Side Shuffle, 3 Sets

60 Second Squat Kickback, alternating sides, 3 Sets

30 Second Side Plank with Hip Abduction, 3 Sets each side

45 Second Inchworm, 3 Sets

45 Second Scissor Skier, 3 Sets

45 Second Crab Kicks, alternating sides, 3 Sets

She Devil

Repeat this circuit of exercise either 3 or 5 times, depending on your skill level. Rest for no more than 2 minutes between each set.

To Failure Tricep Dips

40 Punches

20 Lunge Punches

20 Plank Back Kicks, alternating legs

20 Bridges

10 Raised Leg Bridges

10 Sit-up Punches

10 Clamshells, each side

10 Sitting Twists

Gladiator

Perform this circuit three or five times, depending on your skill level. Avoid resting between exercises, and rest for no more than two minutes between sets.

40 lunges

20 jumping lunges

20 Squats

20 Shoulder taps

40 Mountain Climbers

10 Pushups

10 Up and Down Planks

Full Body Cardio

For these exercises, do two sets of each exercise before moving on. Rest only 30 seconds between each different exercise.

15 Superman

45 Second Single Leg Glute Bridge

45 Second Bicycle Crunches

15 Alternating Squat Jumps

15 Flutter Kicks

15 High Box Jump

15 Judo Pushups

60 Second Burpees

15 Walking Lunges

45 Plank Jacks

45 Second Mountain Climbers

15 Squats

Wake Up Workout

For this circuit, do four to five sets, depending on your skill level. Rest for a minute between each set.

10 Burpees

15 Pushups

20 Mountain Climbers

30 Bicycle Crunches

45 Second Plank

Refresh

These bodyweight exercises should be repeated three times with a minute rest between sets.

15 Lunges

15 Squats

30 Second Wall Squat

60 Second Plank

20 Russian Twists

20 Jumping Jacks

Extreme Arms

For this workout, pick a number of reps you need to feel challenged, but make sure it's not so hard that you have to take a lot of rests. You will do a total of five rounds with a minute rest between exercises and two minutes between sets.

Sets One and Three

10 Forearm Pushups

10 Chin ups

15 Diamond Pushups

Sets Two and Four

10 Dips

10 to 15 Horizontal Pull Ups, elevated feet, and supinated grip

Max out Horizontal Pull Up Hold, you should be able to hold it for at least 10 seconds

Set Five

Max out Dead Hang

Level Six

For this workout, if you find one set easy, do two sets. If that's still too easy, add more sets or try one of the harder workouts in this book.

50 Jumping Jacks

15 Squats

15 Lunges, each leg

60 Russian Twists

25 Vertical Leg Crunches

10 Burpees

10 Oblique Crunches, each side

35 Jumping Jacks

15 V-Ups

15 Tricep Dips

20 Standing Calf Raises

5 Jump Squats

10 Kneeling Pushups

30 Second Plank

Power of 10

This one is pretty self explanatory. There is no need to do more than one set unless this one seems easy.

100 Jumping Jacks

90 Knee Raises

80 Calf Raises

70 Side Lunge

60 Crunches

50 Lunges

40 Side to Side Shuffle

30 Squats

20 Pushups

10 Burpees

3 X 100

Do only one set of this workout.

100 Mountain Climbers

90 Crunches

80 Lunges

70 Donkey Kicks

60Pushups

50 Mountain Climbers

40 Crunches

30 Lunges

20 Donkey Kicks

10 Minute Run

Ultimate

Perform four sets of this exercise. Rest for a couple of minutes between sets and 45 seconds between exercises.

25 Tricep Dips

20 Knee Raises

15 Pull Ups

25 Squats, alternating legs

20 Pushups

15 Decline Pushups

25 Calf Raises, each leg

15 Close Grip Chin Ups

Level Four

This exercise is perfect with just one set, but if you want a little more of a challenge do two sets.

35 Jumping Jacks

10 Tricep Dips

15 Squats

5 Knee Push Ups

10 Calf Raises

35 Russian Twists

30 Second Plank

10 Second Side Plank, each side

30 Jumping Jacks

5 Jump Squats

5 Knee Pushups

5 Burpees

10 to 1

This is a pyramid workout. Begin by doing 10 reps of each exercise, and then start over and 9, 8, 7, and so on until you reach 1.

Mountain Climbers

Touchdowns, alternating hands

Shoulder Taps, alternating hands

Squat Jumps

Speed Skaters

Pushups

Plank jacks

Muffin Top

For this workout, you will do three sets of each exercise and rest for a minute before moving onto the next exercise.

60 Second Run in Place

45 Second Bicycle Crunches

45 Second Dead Bug

60 Second Standing Criss Cross Crunches

30 Second Side Plank Hip Lifts, each side

45 Second Superman

45 Second Inchworm

30 Second Side Bends, each side

45 Second Russian Twist

30 Second Plank

CHAPTER 6

ADVANCED

We've covered a lot of bodyweight exercise moves and benefits, but we have one more thing to look at. Many people believe that the only way to build muscles is by lifting weight, so let's break that myth right now.

Bodyweight training is an amazing way to build muscle. There are plenty of people out there who would argue with you about that, and say only free weights can. A great thing about bodyweight workouts is that they don't hurt your joints like traditional weight training sometimes does. You have a natural motion range and this helps to improve your athleticism overall.

When performing advanced exercises, it requires an unmatched level of tension in the whole body. This is where you get the amazing strength gain. Even still, you will find people that believe that bodyweight training can't be as effective traditional weight training when you are interested in building muscle. This is because it is typically associated with the military, endurance, and high reps. But take a look at the upper body of several male gymnasts, and you get a very different picture.

The main reason why people don't have success with bodyweight workouts is because they don't utilize or know the proper way of bodyweight progressions. That leaves them never increasing their resistance.

They are stuck doing the basic versions of inverted rows and pushups and then start thinking it's too easy for it to be building muscles. And they're not wrong. The basic forms of bodyweight exercises are going to be too easy after awhile and won't provide the amount of tension or overload so that you can build muscles.

Now, what if you started working yourself up to one-armed pushups, one-armed inverted rows, or steep incline pushups? Or you're doing a wide grip inverted row to the neck while your elbows are flared with a two to three-second hold at the top. Then you get so good that you start piling on weighted vests or chains. At that point, it's not a strict bodyweight workout anymore. At that point, it's bodyweight and resistance.

Even still, it is a variation of bodyweight exercises, and it is very effective

One of the other reasons why people think weight training is easier to build muscles is because they can progress by grabbing a heavier weight which is easier than progressing from a frog or cow stand to a planche pushup during the next 18 to 24 months.

You have to have a lot of discipline and patience. Another problem is that while you are gaining muscles and weight with proper nutrition, your bodyweight exercises will become increasingly difficult, preventing you from progressing as quickly. Or you think you aren't progressing as you should, so you give up.

Most trainers out there will tell you that a chin up is better than a pull down when you want to build muscles. Then why are other bodyweight exercises not seen as effective?

Why is a forward lean on a ring dip not seen as effective as a bench press?

Why aren't glute raises just as effective as a leg curl?

I'll argue that they are just as effective. Lack of knowledge about how bodyweight training works and how to progress properly is the main reason why people don't see the results that they want.

You can actually gain muscles quickly if you constantly progress your movements. If you just do several reps, like a lot of people do, that isn't going to help you build muscles.

In order to gain strength and muscle, you have to have a significant amount of load and tension. High reps won't give you either.

You have to activate the fast-twitch fibers in your muscles to build muscles. For the upper body, it's best, if your goal is building muscle, to stick with 5 to 12 repetitions with more advanced moves.

When you are working on the lower body, it's okay to go with higher reps to build muscle. 20 reps of pistol squats on each leg are going to create great leg growth.

Once you cover both of those factors, you have to start adding in the right amount of frequency and volume so that you elicit the strength and muscle gains.

Advanced Moves

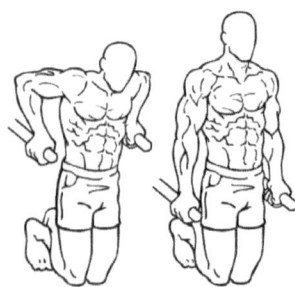

Dips: dips have several variations. For exercises that call for only dips, to perform these you will need a dip bar. Grip the two bars with your elbows bent above the bars. Push yourself up until your elbows lock and then lower back down. To work your chest, angle yourself forward slightly until you feel a pull in your chest. For a straight bar dip, you will use a straight bar positioned at about bellybutton height, and push yourself up and down.

Decline Pushups: This is just like a regular pushup, all you have to do is place your feet on an elevated surface.

Diamond Pushups: Another variation of the regular pushup. Place your hands together to form a diamond shape under the center of your chest and perform pushups as you normally would.

Arching Pushups: For this pushup variation, your hips should be lowered closer to the ground, and your feet should be positioned slightly wider than hip width apartment.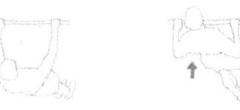

Australian Chin Ups: For this variation on the chin up, you will lower yourself under a straight bar with your feet stretched out in front and your heels on the ground.

In and Out Squat Jumps: This is just like a regular squat jump except your alternate from your feet being together and your feet being open.

Pyramid Calf Raises: These are regular one leg calf raises except you have to complete a pyramid of reps. Meaning, if it says 15 then you would start by doing 15 reps on one leg, rest a couple of seconds, and then do 14 reps on the same leg and continue until you reach one, then repeat on the other leg.

Hannibal Squats: These are regular squats but with your feet together.

Pistol Squats: These are one-legged squats. You squat down on one leg and allow the other to stretch out in front of you; make sure it doesn't touch the ground.

Star Jumps: Begin by standing with your feet hip width apart and your arms by your side. Squat slightly and jump up as high as you can; spreading your legs as wide as they can go and reaching your arms up and out. Come back down to neutral and repeat.

Glute Squeezes: These are super simple. Lay face down with your legs slightly wider than hip width apart. Squeeze your glute muscles and raise your legs as high as you can, keeping your upper body on the ground.

Scissor Chops: Standing, raise your arms straight out in front of you, palms facing each other. Begin making a chopping motion with your arms as fast as you can.

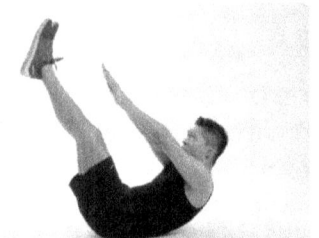

Arm Scissors: Standing, raise your arms straight out in front of you, palms facing down. Start swinging your arms across your body; alternating which arm is on top and which is on bottom.

Side V Crunches: This works like a regular V-up except you are on your side. Begin by lying on your side, the bottom arm extended in front and the other hand behind your head. Using your side muscles, pull your knees and upper elbow towards each other.

Spiderman Planks: Begin in a full plank position and bring your knee out to a 90 degree angle to touch your elbow. Bring that foot back down and repeat with the other leg.

Lying Knee Tucks and Hugs: For tucks, begin by lying flat on you back and engage your abdominal muscles to bring your knees up to your chest. For hugs, begin just like with the tucks, but when you bring you knees in, wrap your arms around them and bring your nose up to touch your knees.

CHAPTER 7

ADVANCED EXERCISES

The following are all advanced exercise routines. There will be a combination of all the previous exercises as well as harder movements. The important thing here is to make sure that you feel challenged. If the number of reps I have listed is easy for you to do, then up the number of reps, or make a move a little harder. Above all else, listen to your body.

Chest Insanity

Perform four sets of these exercises, resting two minutes between each set. You can stop there, or you can move into another isolation routine for the back or legs.

10 straight bar dips

10 decline push ups

10 arching push ups

10 dips

5 diamond push ups

15 regular push ups

Back Brutality

Perform three sets of these exercises, resting two minutes between each set.

5 Upside Down Pull Ups

5 Shoulder Width Pull Ups, behind the neck

5 Wide Grip Pull Ups, behind the neck

5 Close Grip Pull Ups

10 Wide Pull Ups

Arm Assassin

Perform five sets of these exercises, resting two minutes between each set.

20 Tricep Dips

10 Straight Bar Dips

20 Close Grip Australian Chin Ups

10 Close Grip Chin Ups

20 Tricep Dips

10 Dips

20 Wide Grip Australian Chin Ups

10 Shoulder Width Chin Ups

Leg Shocker Routine

Perform five sets of these exercises, resting two minutes between each set.

1 minute Wall Sit

20 Walking Lunges

20 In and Out Squat Jumps

15 Pyramid Calf Raises

20 Hannibal Squats

10 Pistol Squats, per leg

Extreme Full Body

Perform this at least two times. Repeat as many times as you feel you can.

1:30 Jog in Place

15 V-Ups

10 Burpees

30 Russian Twists

10 Pushups

10 Donkey Kicks, per leg

45 Second Plank

10 Burpees

20 Plie Squats

15 Reverse Lunges, per leg

20 Squats

10 Burpees

5 Star Jumps

40 Jumping Jacks

Timer Workout

This workout doesn't count reps. Instead, you will perform a workout for a specific amount of time. For a quick seven minute workout, only perform one set. For a 21 minute workout, perform three sets. Keep track of how many you are able to do in each set, and then compare your numbers the next time you do this workout.

40 Seconds of High Knees, alternating legs

40 Seconds of Burpees

40 Seconds of Plank Jacks

40 Seconds of V-Ups

40 Seconds of Diamond Pushups

40 Seconds of Jump Squats

40 Seconds of Lunge with a Front Kick, alternating legs

40 Seconds of Leg Lifts

40 Seconds of Pistol Squats

40 Seconds of Plank Leg Lifts, alternating legs

300 Workout

This one gets its name because you will be doing 300 reps. There's not need to do more than one set unless you are feeling lucky.

50 Leg Raises

50 Forward Lunges

50 Crunches

50 Tricep Dips

50 Pushups

50 Jump Squats

Summer Booty

Only perform one set of these workouts. Do not rest between each exercise unless you absolutely have to.

10 Single Leg Glute Bridge, each leg

10 Plank Glute Lifts, each leg

10 Wall Squats with Leg Circles, each leg

50 Alternating Curtsy Lunges

50 Alternating Stiff Deadlifts

50 Glue Squeezes

10 Wall Squats with Leg Circles, each leg

10 Plank Glue Lifts, each leg

10 Single Leg Glute Bridge, each leg

Running Strength Workout

Repeat this workout circuit three times. This is great for somebody who is training for a marathon or wants to get into running shape.

¼ Mile Run

15 Squats

¼ Mile Run

10 Pushups

¼ Mile Run

10 Dips

¼ Mile Run

45 Second Plank

Cardio Strength Workout

This is a 15-minute pyramid workout. Only one set is needed. If this is a little too easy for you, start by lowering your squats, choosing a harder pushup variation, and add in 3 burpees after each set of pushups.

1 Sumo Squat	6 Sumo Squats
10 Pushups	5 Pushups
2 Sumo Squats	7 Sumo Squats
9 Pushups	4 Pushups
3 Sumo Squats	8 Sumo Squats
8 Pushups	3 Pushups
4 Sumo Squats	9 Sumo Squats
7 Pushups	2 Pushups
5 Sumo Squats	10 Sumo Squats
6 Pushups	1 Pushups

Explosive Cardio

Begin by completing three sets of circuit one, rest for a minute, and then complete three sets of circuit two. If 60 seconds and three sets are too easy, increase the time to 90 seconds and four sets.

Circuit One

60 Second Forearm Side Plank, repeat on another side

60 Second Mountain Climbers

60 Second Burpees

Circuit Two

60 Second Jump Squats

60 Second Squats

60 Second Jumping Lunges, alternating sides

60 Second Lunges, alternating sides

Cardio HIIT

For this workout, you will be doing an exercise as quickly as you can for 20 seconds then resting for 10 before moving onto the next exercise. Depending on your skill level you can do 5, 7, or 10 sets. Rest for two minutes between each set.

20 Second High Knees

20 Second Punches

20 Second Plank with Jab Cross

20 Second High Knees

20 Second Punches

20 Second Plank Jack with Jab Cross

Do a pushup between each exercise

Power HIIT

For this one, like the last, you can choose between 5, 7, or 10 sets depending on your skill level. Rest for two minutes between each set.

20 Second Squats

20 Second Plank Walk-Outs

20 Second Scissor Chops

20 Second Squats

20 Second Pushups

20 Second Arm Scissors

Do a squat jump between each exercise.

Crazy Legs

There are four circuits in this workout. You will do four rounds of each circuit with minimal rest between each set. Rest for a minute between each circuit.

Circuit One

    20 Second Mountain Climbers

    10 Second Rest

    20 Second Pushups

    10 Second Rest

Circuit Two

    20 Second Side Lunge

    10 Second Rest

    20 Second Squats

    10 Second rest

Circuit Three

    20 Second High Knees

    10 Second Rest

    20 Second Jumping Jacks

    10 Second Rest

Circuit Four

    20 Second Burpees

    10 Second Rest

    20 Second Flutter Kicks

    10 Second Rest

High Energy

For this one, rest for 30 seconds between each circuit. You only have to do one set, but if this feels to easy, start adding more sets until it becomes a challenge.

Circuit One

　10 Crunches

　10 Squats

　10 Jumping Jacks

Circuit Two

　30 Second Plank

　7 Pushups

　25 High Knees, one rep equals two knee raises

Circuit Three

　12 Crunches

　10 Lunges, each leg

　7 Burpees

Circuit Four

　30 Second Plank

　12 Dips

　25 Jumping Jacks

Circuit Five

　12 Crunches

　15 Squats

　25 High Knees

Circuit Six

> 30 Second Plank
>
> 5 Pushups
>
> 10 Burpees

Core Blast

Do the following exercise with no rest. Do two sets with a minute rest between sets.

> 50 Scissor Kicks
>
> 15 Knee Hugs
>
> 50 Windshield Wipers
>
> 15 Lying Knee Tucks
>
> 50 Elbow Plank Butt Ups
>
> 15 Left Side V Crunches
>
> 50 Spiderman Planks, alternating legs
>
> 15 Right Side V Crunches

Conclusion

Thank you for making it through to the end of *Bodyweight Training.* Let's hope it was informative and able to provide you with all of the tools you need to achieve your goals of starting a bodyweight training routine.

The next step is to start using what you have learned. Decide whether you're a beginner, intermediate, or advanced and pick a few of the routines given in this book. All it takes is at least three workouts each week.

Finally, if you found this book useful in any way, a review on Amazon is always appreciated!

Description

Are you tired of shelling out money each month for a gym membership, yet seeing no results? Are you new to exercising and you're looking for someplace to start? Or are you just tired of your old workout plan and you want something new?

If you answered yes to any of these questions, then this book is all you need. Bodyweight training is a perfect place to start for a beginner or an experienced weight trainer. Bodyweight workouts are perfect because they can be performed anywhere and there is no need for any expensive equipment.

Many people still stand by the belief that only lifting weights will give you large muscles, but this book is here to prove them wrong. This book will cover:

- The benefits of bodyweight exercises

- Beginner, intermediate, and advanced exercise routines

- How to perform the exercises

- And much more

These are great exercises to get started and uncover the body you have always dreamed of. By getting this book, you can get started today with your new workout routine.

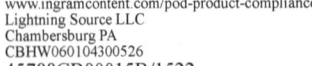